# IMPROVING EYE DISEASE IN 30 DAYS

Reduce Your Risk of Eye Disease in 30 Days:
Macular Degeneration, Retinitis Pigmentosa,
and Diabetic Retinopathy Rehabilitation

## By Robert Redfern

# About the Author

Your Personal Health Coach
www.MyGoodHealthClub.com

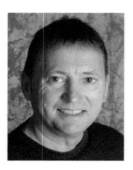

Robert Redfern was born in January 1946. He has helped thousands of people to date in more than 24 countries by providing online health guidance and resources in books, radio interviews, and TV interviews to share his nutritional discoveries. His new book series starts with *Improving Lung Health in 30 Days* and is designed to bring all of his health knowledge into one user-friendly format that anyone can understand when pursuing health recovery.

Robert became interested in health when he and his wife Anne began to take charge of their lifestyle in the late 80s. Robert had not paid much attention to his health until 1986, despite Anne's loving influence. It wasn't until Robert's parents Alfred and Marjorie died prematurely in their 60s that he was forced to re-examine his lifestyle choices.

Robert and Anne embraced a new health philosophy as they examined the health community, medical treatments, and common health issues. After researching the root cause of disease, they discovered that diet and lifestyle choices were the two most pivotal factors that contribute to overall health and wellbeing. Robert and Anne decided to make major changes in their diet and lifestyle, while utilizing **HealthPoint**™ acupressure. The changes that they saw were exceptional.

*In addition to improved health, Robert and Anne both look and feel like they have more vitality than they did decades before they started their new health plan. Currently, Robert, 69, and Anne continue to make healthy choices to live energetically and youthfully, based on a foundation of Natural Health.*

ROBERT REDFERN: YOUR PERSONAL HEALTH COACH
Provides step-by-step guidance on:

# Eye Disease:
## Macular Degeneration, Retinitis Pigmentosa, and Diabetic Retinopathy Rehabilitation in 30 Days

## The Causes and the Recovery Plan

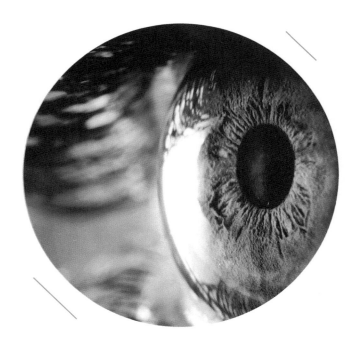

**Publisher:**

**Naturally Healthy Publications. All rights reserved.**

Publication printed in the United Kingdom.

**Publisher's Note:**

This book is not intended to diagnose any disease or offer medical advice. The intention of the book is only to provide information for the reader so that they can make healthy lifestyle choices.

**Warning:**

Some of the information in this book may contradict advice from your physician; nonetheless, content is based on the science of natural health.

# CONTENTS

# Your Commitment Plan to Better Eye Health

| TODAY | I DID THIS | SIGNED I DATE |
|---|---|---|
| I Committed | To regaining and maintaining my eye health for the rest of my life. | |
| I Committed | To drinking 6-8 glasses of water per day with a pinch of sodium bicarbonate in each glass. | |
| I Committed | To spending time in the sun for 20 minutes each day (except when not advised). | |
| I Read | Robert's *Improving Eye Disease in 30 Days* Book. | |
| I Ordered | The recommended supplements to support my plan and healing. | |
| I Planned | My Daily Menu with **ReallyHealthyFoods.com.** | |
| I Started | My breathing exercises. | |
| I Started | Massaging the appropriate acupressure points. | |
| I Reread | Robert's *Improving Eye Disease in 30 Days* Book. | |
| I Reviewed | The recommended supplements to support my plan and healing. | |
| I Reviewed | My water intake. | |
| I Reviewed | My Daily Menu. | |
| I Reviewed | My breathing exercises. | |
| I Reviewed | My life-giving sun exposure (except when not advised). | |
| I Reviewed | How to massage the appropriate acupressure points. | |
| I Recommitted | To regaining and maintaining my eye health for the rest of my life. | |
| I Recommitted | To reading Robert's *Improving Eye Disease in 30 Days* Book. | |
| I Recommitted | To the recommended supplements to support my plan and healing. | |
| I Recommitted | To my water intake. | |
| I Recommitted | To following my Daily Menu. | |
| I Recommitted | To doing my breathing exercises. | |
| I Recommitted | To life-giving sun exposure (except when not advised). | |
| I Recommitted | To massaging the appropriate acupressure points. | |

# Are You Afraid of Losing Your Sight as You Age?

One of the scariest things that can happen as you get older is not spotting that first wrinkle. It is realizing that your vision may be on the decline.

According to a recent survey of 2000 British adults from ages 30 to 60, conducted by eye care specialists Bausch + Lomb and commissioned by Ocuvite, 42 percent of people think that deteriorating eyesight is inevitable.

 *How frightening.*

There's more. All survey participants from 11 different countries, encompassing 11,000 people in China, Germany, France, Brazil, India, Japan, Italy, Russia, Spain, the US, and the UK , revealed that they would give up almost anything to keep their vision. Bausch + Lomb researchers believe that this response confirms that sight may be our **most valuable sense.**

Yet these same survey participants had no idea how to protect their eyes to prevent vision loss in the future. Though 79 percent of participants would rather give up their hearing, or even a limb at 68 percent, rather than lose their sight, there was very little understanding of how to sustain long-term eye health.

*The eyes are the window into your soul, and they are also a strong indicator of your future.*

If your vision has declined and continues to weaken, so will your quality of life. If you are already affected by eye disease, all hope is not lost. In this book, we will explore a complete rehabilitation plan for eye disease recovery, based on lifestyle changes and essential nutrients that can transform your health.

If you fear losing your sight with age, this is the book you have been waiting for. No matter how old or how young you may be, this plan can make a difference. After recently helping an acquaintance named Ethel, age 99, recover her eyesight damaged by wet age-related macular degeneration, I am a believer. Ethel overcame this so-called "normal" side effect of aging, caused primarily by malnutrition. Her vision is steadily improving.

*"Doing nothing is not an option for those who value their independence and who want to maintain their quality of life. If your doctor disagrees with the current scientific research and does not support your efforts, then you will need to seek the help of EyeSight Action (Eyesight.nu) or a more sympathetic professional."*

*- Focus On Saving Eyesight, Naturally Healthy Publications*

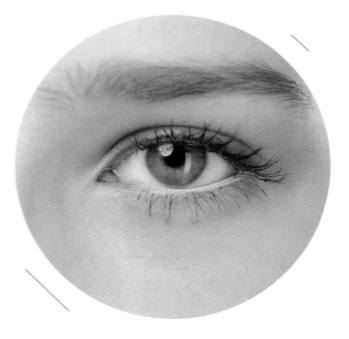

# Why Is Your Eyesight at Risk?

When you visit your optometrist, you may be told that there is no known cause of eye disease. Sadly, many conventional eye doctors have little to no training in nutrition. They may provide no hope for vision decline. However, a different group of doctors and researchers have uncovered important information that can change the way you see the world.

## Everything Is Crystal Clear

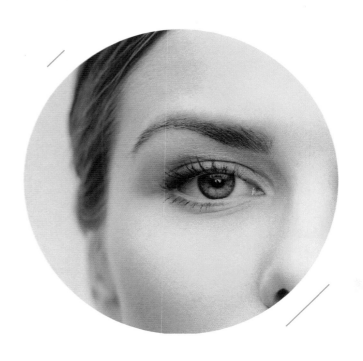 *Eye diseases are caused by, or worsened by, malnutrition and nutritional deficiencies.*

**Here are the nutrients you need every day for clear vision and vibrant health:**

- Proteins, fats, and carbohydrates
- Roughly 13 vitamins
- 20-60 minerals, depending on which scientist you believe
- Roughly 12 amino acids
- Roughly 10 essential fatty acids
- Roughly 6 digestive enzymes, from plants
- Oxygen
- Pure water
- Probiotics, the healthy bacteria found in your gut

On this list of important nutrients, you can't have one without the other. These nutrients work as cofactors. A deficiency in one will cause malnutrition across-the-board. To provide a better example, there are more than 80 enzymes at work in your body as we speak that require zinc as a critical cofactor.

Most of us do not eat enough of the nutrients we need to protect our eyes each day. Even worse, your body may not be prepared to *absorb* these nutrients when you do eat them, because of age and because of existing inflammation caused by an un-natural diet. If you want to protect your vision, time is not on your side. Research confirms that the average 70-year-old has only 20 percent of the beneficial enzymes needed for digestion compared to that of a 20-year-old.

*"Over 45? Having an eye test at least once every two years should be part of everyone's healthcare routine. Many causes of sight loss are preventable if they are caught early with nutritional changes."*

*- Naturally Healthy News, Issue 27*

It's no wonder that eye disease is on the rise. In this book, you'll discover a step-by-step rehabilitation plan that you can tailor to your eye condition to preserve your sight for the future.

Let's begin...

# Age-Related Macular Degeneration: What Is It?

Age-related macular degeneration affects the macular of the eye, also known as the central part of the retina. ARMD is a progressive disease, meaning it will worsen over time. Around the world, ARMD ranks as the third cause of blindness after cataract and glaucoma, according to the World Health Organization.

👁 *The part of the vision affected by ARMD is called central vision.*

Central vision is the process by which "millions of cells change light into nerve signals that tell the brain what the person is seeing." This affects activities like reading a book and driving a car, in addition to a multitude of other daily tasks.

**ARMD can be categorized in two types:**

1. **Dry** - Changes that don't involve any form of fluid leakage.

2. **Wet** - Usually accompanies dry ARMD; changes involve fluid leaking, e.g., blood, that stems from new blood vessels growing underneath the retina.

*Blindness in the elderly is largely due to ARMD.*

## Who Gets It?

Members of the white, non-Hispanic population have the highest risk of ARMD, while members of the black population have the lowest risk.

## Others at risk include:

- **Members of the older population - 70 and up**
- **Smokers**
- **Those with a family history**
- **Overweight individuals**
- **Nutritionally deficient individuals**

Research at this time is inconclusive; however, high blood pressure and sunlight may contribute to ARMD. Age-related macular degeneration remains one of the main causes of sight loss in those over 50. ARMD is now being diagnosed in younger people because of countless modern lifestyle factors that can damage vision—including staring at a computer all day long, eating un-natural foods, and being exposed to environmental toxins.

*"Remember: Blindness can vary, from minor problems that affect our daily activities, to up to 95 percent sight loss that steals our independence and quality of life. Take your eye health very seriously."*

*- Focus On Saving Eyesight, Naturally Healthy Publications*

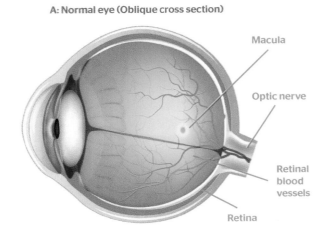

A: Normal eye (Oblique cross section)

Macula
Optic nerve
Retinal blood vessels
Retina

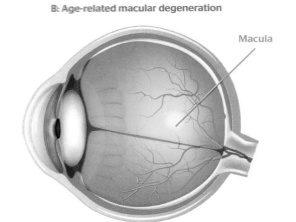

B: Age-related macular degeneration

Macula

*Source: St. Mark's Eye Institute*

## Age-Related Macular Degeneration Signs and Symptoms

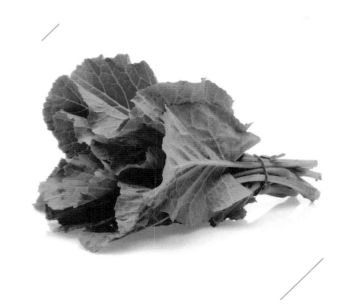 *There are no signs or symptoms in the beginning stages of macular degeneration.*

*"Over 25 epidemiological studies examining dietary intake of carotenoids found that lutein and zeaxanthin are inversely associated with age-related macular degeneration,"* said Andrew Shao, technical services manager for vitamins and dietary supplements at Kemin Foods.

*- Focus On Saving Eyesight, Naturally Healthy Publications*

### When symptoms do appear, they include:

- Loss of central vision
- Altered perception of colors
- Distortion of straight lines

### How Is It Treated?

Certain types of laser treatments are utilized with wet ARMD; however, these treatments are ineffective for dry ARMD. Surgery is also not an option for dry ARMD. Surgeries for wet ARMD are available but not recommended due to the complications involved.

### What Causes It?

### ARMD Dietary Factors

In addition to an overall anti-inflammatory diet and lifestyle (exercise also lowers risk), certain nutrients and dietary factors are associated with the prevention and progression of ARMD.

### Foods and nutrients that decrease the risk of ARMD include:

- Beta-carotene
- Fruits
- Primary carotenoids lutein and zeaxanthin – Offer over 40 percent decreased risk, with collard greens and spinach providing the most protection
- Vitamins C and E
- Vegetables (dark leafy greens)
- Zinc

### Foods that increase the risk of ARMD include:

- Those high in saturated fat and cholesterol
- Processed foods and baked goods - Double the risk of ARMD, as well as increasing blood lipids and inflammation in the body

The visual effects of ARMD...

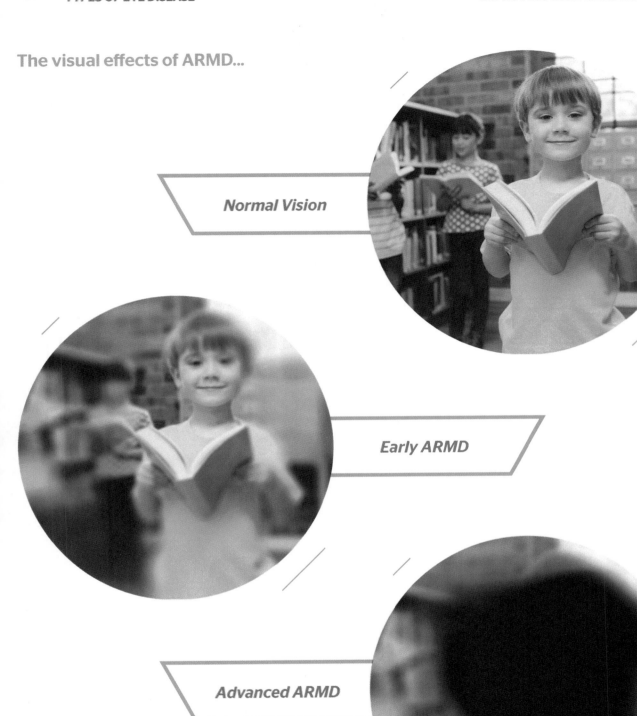

**Normal Vision**

**Early ARMD**

**Advanced ARMD**

# Retinitis Pigmentosa: What Is It?

Retinitis pigmentosa (RP) is the most well-known genetic eye disease. Many cases of severe eye disease in children, such as microphthalmos (small eye), cataracts, glaucoma in retinoblastoma, and an eye tumor in childhood, are caused by genetic defects.

Retinitis pigmentosa is a group of inherited eye diseases that damage the retina. This layer of tissue found at the back of the inner eye, called the retina, is needed to convert light images to nerve signals that are sent to the brain. As the light-sensitive retina in the eye begins to degenerate as a result of disease, it can cause blindness.

The rare condition affects roughly one in 4000 people. More than 1.5 million people worldwide suffer from RP as it remains the most common hereditary retinal degeneration. Retinitis pigmentosa is the number one cause of inherited blindness in developed countries.

## Who Gets It?

👁 *The first signs of retinitis pigmentosa are usually detected in childhood and may affect both eyes.*

A child may experience poor night vision and a narrowing field of sight. As retinitis pigmentosa advances in the later stages, only a small portion of the central vision will remain with limited peripheral vision. The greatest risk factor for retinitis pigmentosa is family history.

## Common symptoms of RP include:

- Decreased vision in low light or at night
- Tunnel vision, i.e. loss of peripheral vision
- Loss of central vision in later stages

A: Normal eye anatomy
Cornea
Iris
Lens
Pupil
Macula
Fovea
Optic Nerve

B: Retinitis pigmentosa
The retina has pigment deposits known as "bone spicules"

*Source: David A. Steenblock, D.O.*

## How Is It Treated?

There are some aspects of most genetic eye diseases that can be treated, but as yet, treatment to put right the genetic problem itself is not available for these conditions. There is a great deal of research being done into genetic disorders. It is reasonable to expect advances in treatment in future years.

## What Causes It?

Retinitis pigmentosa is an inherited group of diseases without a specific known cause. The eye diseases may be related to 32 different genes that can be passed down through a family. A child is likely to have this dominant genetic trait when a parent has retinitis pigmentosa. Up to one percent of the population may have these genetic markers for retinitis pigmentosa.

Dr. Caldwell B. Esselstyn Jr., a former surgeon at the Cleveland Clinic, President of the Cleveland Clinic staff, author, and researcher, is famous for saying, "Genes load the gun, but lifestyle pulls the trigger."

*This is never more applicable than when it comes to eye disease.*

While genetics do play a role in retinitis pigmentosa, lifestyle choices can influence how genes are expressed or activated. Though medical treatment is limited, retinitis pigmentosa also responds to an alternative treatment for ARMD. The issue stems from a lack of nutritional uptake from within the digestive tract, which prevents the right nutrients from absorbing into the eye.

## The "Miracle" Spice for Retinitis Pigmentosa

Curcumin is a phytochemical and belongs to a class of compounds known as curcuminoids. Other than being an important component of turmeric, a favorite Indian spice, curcumin is a natural polyphenol, a group of chemicals which provide many health benefits. However, turmeric is not curcumin—curcumin is thousands of times more powerful than simple turmeric. Curcumin is a standardized extract from the dried root of the curcuma plant, the root being the portion used for medicinal purposes.

Research now proves why ancient medicine has used curcumin for thousands of years. Even though **curcumin's chemical makeup** was determined in 1910, it took until the mid-1970s and 80s to study curcumin on a large scale.

Sufferers of retinitis pigmentosa have even more reason to pay attention to this ancient root. The National Eye Institute reports, based on the findings of University of California San Diego associate professor of ophthalmology Radha Ayyagari, Ph.D., that curcumin may be used by doctors as a simple alternative to treat common cases of RP.

When researchers gave curcumin to rats with genetically engineered eye problems similar to retinitis pigmentosa, poor electrical responses to light and thinning retinas in the eyes were alleviated. Curcumin preserved the rats' rods and cones in the retina, while increasing light-induced electrical responses in the eye. Study results suggest only positive benefits from using curcumin to address eye problems associated with retinitis pigmentosa.

Dr. Ayyagari concluded, "Coming from India, I have a lot of faith in curcumin."

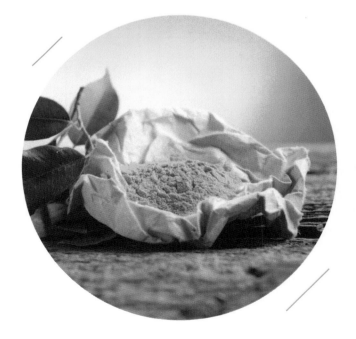

# Diabetic Retinopathy: What Is It?

## There are four stages of diabetic retinopathy:

- **Stage 1:** Mild non-proliferative retinopathy
- **Stage 2:** Moderate non-proliferative retinopathy
- **Stage 3:** Severe non-proliferative retinopathy
- **Stage 4:** Proliferative retinopathy

Diabetic retinopathy is just one of the three eye diseases which are often associated with diabetes. The risk for having cataracts and glaucoma are also increased when diabetes is present. The World Health Organization currently attributes one percent of global blindness to diabetes.

These stages cover the progression of the disease and the changes that result from that progression. These changes range from micro aneurysms in the retina, blockage of the blood vessels that feed the retina, and the growth of abnormal blood vessels, which may leak blood.

👁 *Diabetic retinopathy is the eye disease that occurs most frequently after a diabetes diagnosis.*

Diabetic retinopathy is a primary contributor to blindness for adults in Western countries and is therefore very dangerous. Diabetic retinopathy is characterized by certain changes in the blood vessels of the retina. The retina is defined as "a light-sensitive layer of tissue, lining the inner surface of the eye."

*"Not all eye doctors know (or agree) that nutritional deficiency is the cause of eye problems. If you believe them and do nothing, then you have no chance for recovery. If you give it a fair 12 months trial, you have a good chance for recovery."*

*- Focus On Saving Eyesight, Naturally Healthy Publications*

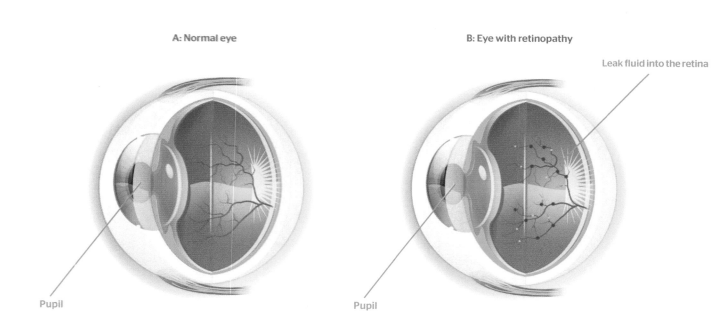

A: Normal eye          B: Eye with retinopathy

Leak fluid into the retina

Pupil          Pupil

*Source: Solomon Eye Associates*

# Who Gets It?

Anyone with type 1 or type 2 diabetes is at risk for eye disease. Almost half of all people living with these types of diabetes have diabetic retinopathy. The vast majority of those diagnosed with diabetes, i.e. 80-90 percent, have type 2 diabetes.

👁 *A diagnosis of type 2 diabetes can be thought of as a precursor to diabetic eye disease.*

Obviously, avoiding diabetes in the first place can eliminate the concern over contracting an eye disease associated with this condition. The fact is that type 2 diabetes is a 100 percent lifestyle condition caused by eating bread, pastry, cookies, breakfast cereal, pizza, white rice, high-sugar foods, potatoes, parsnips, sugary drinks, and pasta. The full Diabetes Rehabilitation Plan can be found in my book, *Solving Diabetes Type 2 in 27 Days*.

## Type 2 Diabetes Risk Factors

*   **Family Diet History** - Increases risk when parents, brothers, sisters, children, grandparents, grandchildren, aunts, uncles, nephews, nieces, or half-siblings eating the same diet have the disease.

*   **Age** - 40 or over is when risk is highest.

*   **Abdominal Obesity** - Too much abdominal fat in the stomach and abdominal area, a.k.a. belly fat or central obesity.

*   **History of Gestational Diabetes**

*   **High Blood Pressure**

*   **High Cholesterol**

*   **Cultural Background** - Black, Latino, American Indian/Alaskan Native, or Asian and Pacific Islander populations (only when eating a high-starch/sugar diet).

*   **Prior Impaired Fasting Glucose** - Or currently impaired glucose tolerance.

## The American Diabetes Association's list of symptoms for type 2 diabetes includes:

*   **Frequent urination**
*   **Unusual thirst**
*   **Extreme hunger**
*   **Unusual weight loss**
*   **Extreme fatigue and irritability**
*   **Frequent infections**
*   **Blurred vision**
*   **Cuts/bruises that are slow to heal**
*   **Tingling/numbness in the hands/feet**
*   **Recurring skin, gum, or bladder infections**

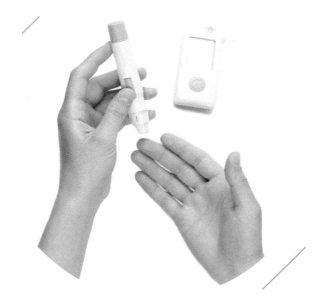

# Diabetic Retinopathy Signs and Symptoms

There may be no symptoms if you have diabetic retinopathy. This is one of the reasons it is so dangerous. If there are symptoms present, they will manifest as blurred vision or floaters in the eyes consisting of spots or blood.

*Diabetics should see a qualified eye doctor at least once a year. If the disease progresses, eye surgery may be necessary.*

## How Is It Treated?

While there is no cure for diabetic retinopathy, some treatment options to manage the condition are available. Your doctor may recommend photocoagulation laser treatment to prevent vision loss before retinal damage has progressed too far. If the retina is not badly damaged, a surgery called a vitrectomy can be used to remove vitreous gel for possible sight improvement.

It is important to understand that diabetic retinopathy treatment is only used to delay or reduce vision loss. Surgical treatment cannot provide the nutrients necessary to rehabilitate eye disease over the long-term.

## What Causes It?

The chronic inflammation which leads to diabetic retinopathy may be due to a number of factors. Some of these factors are the same as those that lead to diabetes, including:

- **Smoking**
- **Elevated cholesterol**
- **High blood pressure**
- **Inattention to controlling blood glucose levels**
- **Length of time diabetes has been present**

*A high-fat, low-fiber diet full of glycotoxins and lacking in enzymes, nutrients, and healthy foods may also contribute to diabetic retinopathy.*

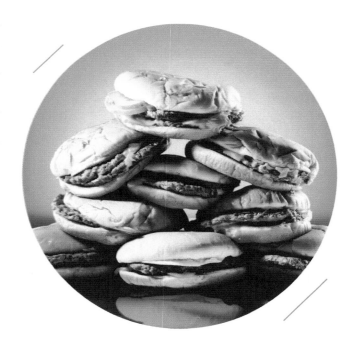

# Glycotoxins, Diabetes, and Your Eyes

What are glycotoxins? Glycotoxins are a byproduct of the glycation process. Glycation is the process by which sugar interacts with proteins and/or certain lipids (fats) in an uncontrolled manner without the presence of enzymes. When foods with the potential for forming glycotoxins are cooked using improper cooking methods, sugars bind non-enzymatically to proteins, resulting in glycotoxins.

## There are two types of glycotoxins:

- **AGEs** - Advanced glycation end products
- **ALEs** - Advanced lipoxidation end products

### 👁 What do glycotoxins have to do with diabetes and the eyes?

These toxins play a role in the complications, including eye disease, associated with having diabetes due to their ability to flourish in blood with elevated sugar levels. While absorption rates of dietary glycotoxins are somewhat low, the excretion rate is even lower—meaning, they are accumulating in body tissues. This is one reason diabetics have complications related to the nerves (neuropathies), kidneys, cardiovascular system, and the eyes, as these are some of the areas accumulation takes place.

## Food, Inflammation, and Glycotoxins

Glycation and the resulting glycotoxins cause an inflammatory response in the body. Too much glucose in the bloodstream for too long and/or choosing foods that are high in glycotoxins leads to inflammation.

The formation of glycotoxins depends upon the choice of foods and the way they are prepared. Cooking foods at temperatures above 250° that are high in protein, fat, or fructose substantially increases the production of glycotoxins.

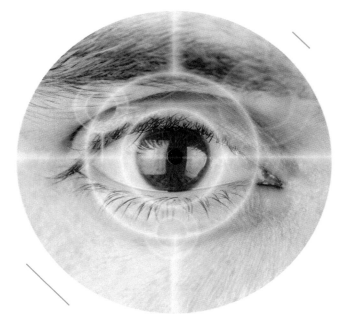

## Cooking methods (liquid) that can decrease the formation of glycotoxins include:

- Steaming
- Poaching
- Braising
- Stewing
- Boiling

## Cooking methods (dry) that can *increase* the formation of glycotoxins include:

- Baking
- Broiling
- Grilling
- Barbequing
- Frying

## While all foods containing protein, fat, and/or fructose have the potential to produce some glycotoxins, certain foods in particular are significant sources of glycotoxins:

- **Foods high in fat *and* protein, i.e., animal products**
- **Foods high in fructose or HFCS**

Other than grilling some pineapple on a rare occasion, what sources of cooked fructose are there? Surprise! Pasteurized juices, including the orange juice you drink every morning, and all those sodas you drink containing high fructose corn syrup (which virtually all do) are good sources of glycotoxins.

*Consumer Beware! Glycotoxins are already present in many other processed foods and have been for years.*

C-reactive protein (CRP), a marker for inflammation in the body, decreases with reducing glycotoxins in the diet. Another marker for inflammation, the cytokine tumor necrosis factor-alpha, *increases* with glycotoxin intake.

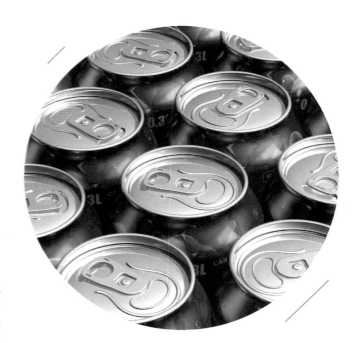

# Are Your Eyes Inflamed?

👁 *Inflammation is the root of all disease (except for gene dysfunction).*

Eye diseases are no exception. Just as inflammation is behind chronic disease (cardiovascular disease, cancer, and, as we have seen, diabetes), it is also behind the manifestation of eye diseases. Inflammation of the eye is a result of many of the same things that create inflammation in other parts of the body.

*"According to estimates, about 25 percent of people over the age of 65 will end up with some form of sight loss."*

*- Naturally Healthy News*

## Free Radicals, Oxidative Stress, and the Inflammation Connection

A healthier diet is higher in antioxidants, the substances that fight off and neutralize free radicals. By definition, free radicals are an atom or group of atoms that have at least one unpaired electron and are therefore unstable and highly reactive. Oxidative stress occurs when the body is exposed to an excessive number of free radicals. Oxidative stress damages the cells, including cellular DNA, proteins, and membranes.

👁 *Simply living creates free radicals, as does exercise and the process of eating and digestion.*

We do require some level of free radicals to function. However, due to our excessive lifestyles of drinking, smoking, and eating toxic foods, our bodies are in overload. Fortunately, antioxidants, available in high-quality foods and supplements, can fight off these free radicals and the damage they do to the body. This includes the inflammation associated with eye disease.

On top of that, eye problems can be caused by nutritional issues, like food intolerances. Food intolerance may result in poor nutrient absorption to contribute to malnutrition in the eyes. A mineral-poor diet caused by natural erosion and over-farming of soil only makes the problem worse.

**A non-inflammatory diet that can protect your vision includes the following foods (except when temporarily contraindicated for recovery):**

- **Any kind of vegetable—focusing on non-starchy vegetables, especially dark leafy greens; yams/ sweet potatoes are fine in moderation.**
- **Legumes; beans, peas, and lentils of all kinds.**
- **Alternative to grains and cereals; quinoa, millet, buckwheat, and other seeds.**
- **Low-sugar, dark-skinned fruits like avocados, blueberries, blackberries, black currants, etc.**
- **Hemp seeds daily.**

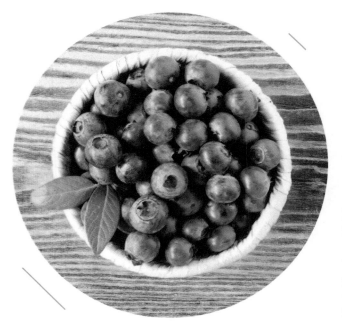

# Your Eyes Are Starving for Nutrition

Did you know that out of every organ in your body, your eyes have the greatest need for nutrients and oxygen? Malnutrition that comes from a depleted, inflammatory diet and poor circulation caused by a lifestyle condition like type 2 diabetes can immediately impact your eye health.

👁 *Even as you get older, eating well may not be enough.*

Essential nutrients may not be well-absorbed with age. This can result in more serious problems, like retinitis pigmentosa. The only way to ensure that the proper nutrients reach your eyes in the shortest amount of time is to focus on the health of your digestive tract. When digestion is optimal, fresh foods and high-quality supplements with the highest bioavailability will reach their intended destination.

## Eyesight Nutrients A to Z

Many of us are familiar with antioxidants proven to benefit vision, like vitamins A, C, E, copper, selenium, and zinc. But today, there are a number of new nutrients on the scene that pack an even more powerful punch—including the amino acid taurine, lutein, curcumin, astaxanthin, and zeaxanthin.

## Considering that our modern soil and food supply are depleted, your eyes need these nutrients more than ever:

- **Astaxanthin:** The red-carotenoid pigment astaxanthin, which gives crustaceans their color, is 65 times more powerful than vitamin C. What's more, astaxanthin is renowned among researchers as a primary supporter of eye health—it is one of the few protective antioxidants able to penetrate the retinal barrier. Astaxanthin supplementation may provide relief for macular degeneration and other eye diseases; researchers noted that the antioxidant accumulated in eye tissue when fed to rats.

- **Curcumin:** Potent curcumin is needed to stimulate the body's production of the essential eye-protective antioxidant glutathione, discussed on the next page. Because of its antioxidant, anti-inflammatory, and anti-carcinogenic effects, researchers consider curcumin to be "a promising drug for the treatment of cancer and retinal diseases." As discussed, curcumin also has beneficial application in the treatment of retinitis pigmentosa.

- **Lutein:** After taking lutein supplements in high doses for two to four weeks, 16 retinitis pigmentosa patients showed improved visual acuity and visual fields; these results were most noticeable in blue-eyed individuals. Scientists have confirmed for more than 20 years that eating foods high in lutein can reduce the risk of macular degeneration. In the Age-Related Eye Disease Study Research Group conducted on 4519 people, researchers concluded that consuming yellow plant pigments lutein and zeaxanthin at higher levels could lower the risk of ARMD.

- **Taurine:** Based on research published in the Alternative Medicine Review, retinitis pigmentosa sufferers may have faulty cellular uptake of the most prolific amino acid in the eye, taurine. RP patients may also have disturbed vitamin A utilization and could benefit from a vitamin A supplement.

- **Zeaxanthin:** Zeaxanthin and astaxanthin sound similar because they are both pigment compound carotenoids that give some bright fruits, vegetables, and seafood their color. As a potent carotenoid antioxidant, zeaxanthin works with lutein to protect the macula from free radical damage often associated with ARMD. As confirmed by Dr. Yeum in 1995, zeaxanthin and lutein are the only two carotenoid antioxidants that can be found in the eye lens and retina. Researchers reported that consuming 6 mg of lutein along with co-nutrient zeaxanthin daily for five months helped to significantly increase macular pigment density, which can protect against harmful blue wavelength light that may be most responsible for macular degeneration.

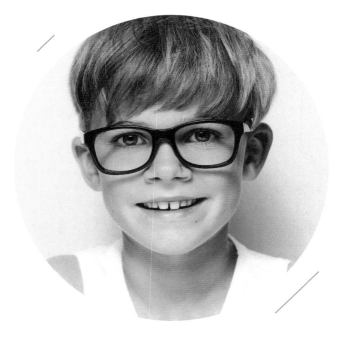

# Glutathione: The All-Star Antioxidant for Your Eyes

One high-quality supplement that holds the key to healthy vision is SAM-e, short for S-adenosyl methionine. SAM-e is a naturally occurring amino acid, present throughout the body, with high levels in the brain, adrenal glands, and liver.

## Where Does Glutathione Fit In?

SAM-e is a source of *glutathione*. Glutathione is present in all cells. It is a powerful primary antioxidant. It protects the body, including the eyes. It is imperative for those with stress and anxiety because these conditions, along with aging and many other factors such as an inflammatory diet and lifestyle, deplete glutathione levels in the body.

*If you could only take one nutritional path to care for your eyes, that path would be lined with glutathione.*

Research shows a strong connection between glutathione and the prevention of diabetic retinopathy, retinitis pigmentosa, and ARMD.

## Why Else Is Glutathione Important?

Glutathione recycles antioxidants, meaning it allows the body to use antioxidants over and over again.

This is a big plus when it comes to regaining overall health and supporting the health of the eyes:

- Glutathione is a detoxifier and transports toxins out of the body, including glycotoxins.
- Glutathione increases immune function and controls inflammation.
- Glutathione protects the cells and enhances energy metabolism.
- The chronically ill have been found to have very low levels of glutathione. This finding supports the need for glutathione in the prevention of disease.

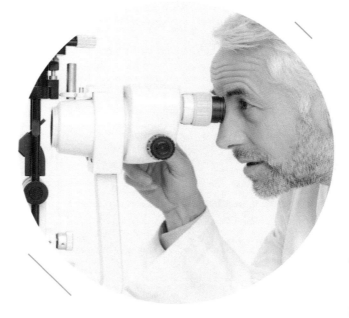

## Glutathione as a Supplement

*Since glutathione is obviously so important, why not just take a glutathione supplement instead of taking SAM-e?*

Taking SAM-e is critical because **glutathione can't be taken directly**. It will not survive the digestive process; however, it can be utilized when taken in another form through what is called a precursor. A precursor by definition is: a substance, cell, or cellular component from which another substance, cell, or cellular component is formed. In this case, SAM-e!

Glutathione is also available in a healthy, non-inflammatory diet or through other high-quality precursors.

### Foods that make up a healthy diet and boost glutathione levels at the same time include:

- **Asparagus**
- **Cruciferous vegetables** - Broccoli, dark leafy greens, cabbage, cauliflower
- **Garlic**
- **Onion**

### Other high-quality precursors to glutathione are:

- **Alpha lipoic acid R**
- **B vitamins** - Folate, B6, B12 (methylcobalamin)
- **Milk thistle**
- **N-acetyl-cysteine**
- **The trace mineral selenium**
- **Vitamins C and E** (in the form of mixed tocopherols)

*Engaging in the proper exercise can also elevate glutathione levels in the body.*

SAM-e is derived from the amino acid methionine. SAM-e is produced when methionine and adenosine triphosphate, better known as ATP, are combined. SAM-e is only secondary to ATP as the ultimate energy molecule since SAM-e is also a methyl donor and is involved in a process called methylation. Methylation assists the body in protecting itself from cellular damage, premature aging, brain dysfunction, and many other chronic diseases, including diabetes and eye disease.

A simple change in lifestyle and supplementing with essential, well-researched nutrients, including SAM-e, may spare you and your loved ones a slow decline in vision. These powerful nutrients support eye health and overall wellbeing to reduce the risk of chronic disease.

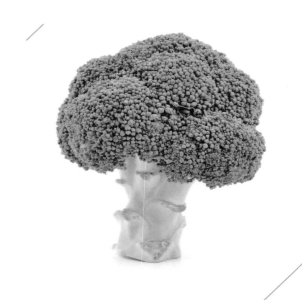

# The Western Un-Natural Food Diet

Nutritional therapy in the form of an anti-inflammatory diet and the appropriate supplements is crucial in strengthening the immune system, decreasing inflammation, and winning the battle against eye disease. A diet that will definitely hinder your prevention and recovery is the Western Un-Natural Food Diet.

👁 *Nothing affects us more than what we choose to eat at least three to four times a day, every day.*

Most of us lack the essential nutrients in our diet needed for good health, perpetuating inflammation. These nutrients include selenium, iodine, magnesium, B vitamins, chromium, and others. These factors combined with one or more poor choices are part of a disease-promoting lifestyle.

The "Balanced Western Diet" (now better described as the Western Un-Natural Food Diet) is the number one disease-promoting and inflammation-producing diet in modern society. It is consumed more and more on a daily basis.

This highly inflammatory diet is made up of sugary foods in the form of breads, pastas, cereals, and potatoes. The Western Un-Natural Food Diet is way too high in unhealthy fats and lacks the antioxidants and phytochemicals your body needs to eliminate free radicals. This all-too-common diet is lacking in high-fiber foods and the foods that provide essential nutrients necessary to find relief from eye disease—and to prevent it in the first place.

## These missing foods include:

- **Beans** (except when temporarily contraindicated for recovery)
- **Dark-skinned fruits**
- **Nuts**
- **Seeds**
- **Vegetables** (especially broccoli and kale)

*"Research shows common eye disorders can be slowed and even reversed using the appropriate nutrition."*

*- Naturally Healthy News, Issue 21*

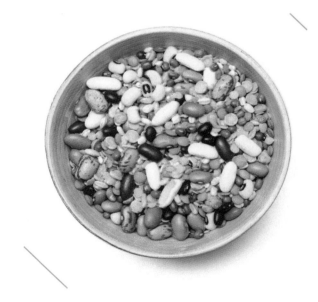

# Can I Reverse Eye Disease?

I prefer not to use the word "cure" when talking about these health conditions since many cases are directly related or exacerbated by lifestyle factors.

Cure is a popular medical buzzword, although the medical field cannot provide cures. (Many people argue that this is on purpose since it would put Big Pharma out of business.) Every health condition has a cause. When you take away the underlying cause and follow a non-inflammatory lifestyle, your body will have the support it needs to repair itself, in many cases.

When you remove the cause and support your body with healthy lifestyle choices and nutrients, you can often grow healthy again. You may call this a cure, but I believe it to be making healthy lifestyle choices.

Since these health conditions are inflammatory, a non-inflammatory lifestyle is a must. It's important to stay hydrated by drinking six to eight 16 ounce (500 ml) glasses of pure, clean water per day. You can heal your body with vital nutrients and antioxidants found in vitamins, minerals, healthy carbohydrates, amino acids, and essential fatty acids.

## Optimal Nutritional Management

Optimal nutritional management is essential for the repair of damaged tissues, for the reduction of inflammation, and for the quality, as well as the length, of life.

Did you know those who consider themselves happy have less inflammation than those who don't? It could certainly be argued that a well-rested person who is of a healthy weight; limits toxins; focuses on a diet bountiful in foods which are nourishing, anti-inflammatory, and a source of enzymes and antioxidants; and who also supplements with high-quality nutrients is an individual who is happy indeed!

*Healing starts with nutritional therapy.*

*Detoxification may be uncomfortable at first, but this too will pass.*

*Sensible eating can support your recovery.*

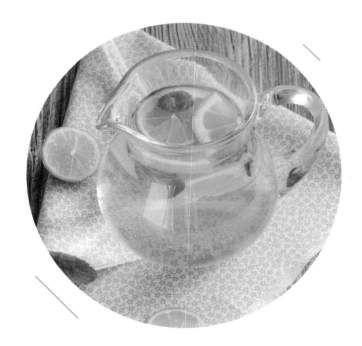

*...transform your health with a balanced lifestyle and essential nutrients...*

# The Nutrients You Need

**Studies show the following high-quality nutrients can prevent, slow down, or even reverse the eye diseases discussed in this book:**

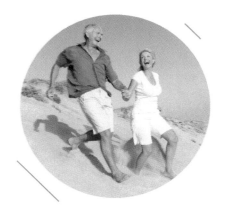

- **Lutein, Zeaxanthin Extract, L-Taurine, Bilberry Extract, and 22 Vitamins and Minerals** - High levels of key carotenoids lutein and zeaxanthin have been shown to be essential for eye health.

- **Krill Oil or Hemp Seed Oil (vegetarian alternative)** - Contains concentrated Omega 3, 6, and 9 oils that can stabilize blood sugar levels and provide protection for cell membranes, amongst other health benefits; can boost the immune system and support a positive mental state.

- **Astaxanthin** - Powerful biological antioxidant that provides support for healthy eyes.

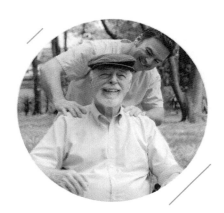

- **90 Vitamins, Minerals, and Nutrients** - Deliver a full spectrum of liquid, highly-absorbable multivitamins and minerals.

- **Taurine** - Can support the delivery of nutrients into the retinal cells and reduce oxidative damage to the eyes.

- **Vitamin C** - Provides powerful support to increase energy and maintain the protein collagen of tissues, helping them to heal.

- **Serrapeptase, Curcumin, Ecklonia Cava Extract, and Vitamin D3** - Clears inflammation and encourages healthy blood flow and circulation to the eyes.

- **Alpha Lipoic Acid** - Supports eye health and repairs oxidative damage, regenerating other antioxidants.

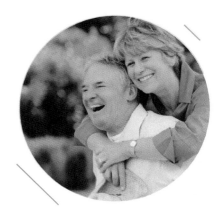

# What If My Doctor Doesn't Support My Recovery?

You can use this Eye Disease Rehabilitation Program to improve your health alongside any medical treatment and still get the benefits! Your doctor has an obligation to stick with the prescription drug outline that fits into the pharmaceutical industry monopoly. This includes the AMA in the US and the GMC in the UK.

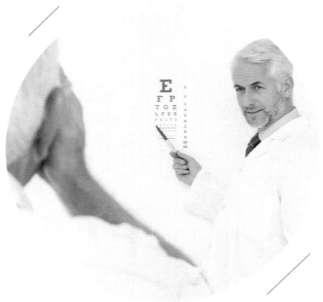

Make no mistake—these organizations make money off disease care for sick individuals. They don't have a business model that promotes actual health recovery in any way, shape, or form. These organizations push a patented prescription drug protocol that allows them to charge outrageous prices for drug use over a lifetime. At the very best, these drugs may help the patient to feel better, but in many scenarios, they could lead to their death.

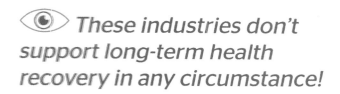 *These industries don't support long-term health recovery in any circumstance!*

These organizations are protected by the FDA in the US and the MHRA in the UK. They receive backing from powerful political parties and politicians who continue to fund the disease care monopoly I have just described.

*Yet when you follow the Eye Disease Rehabilitation Program to the letter, you may start to see results within 30 days.*

It will be a good day when drug companies are totally banned from contacting or influencing doctors, both directly and indirectly. It will be a good day when the information doctors need to prescribe drugs is made available from an independent body with a legal responsibility to ensure the efficacy and safety of drugs.

# Your Eye Disease Rehabilitation Plan

## 10 Steps for Long-Term Health Recovery

This self-recovery protocol can be used by sufferers of eye disease
and to support long-term eye health, in most cases:

| | | | |
|---|---|---|---|
| 1 | Clear inflammation and facilitate healing | Eat really healthy foods | 6 |
| 2 | Supplement missing nutrients | Stay active daily | 7 |
| 3 | Boost the immune system | Learn proper breathing | 8 |
| 4 | Drink more water | Stimulate acupressure points | 9 |
| 5 | Cut out un-natural, high-sugar foods | Get more sun exposure | 10 |

It's almost impossible *not* to see significant health changes after applying many of the points in this 10 Step Plan.
You can clear up numerous symptoms and may see a full recovery, in many cases.

For details of the suggested plans, turn to **page 39.**

# 1. Clear Inflammation and Facilitate Healing

- **MaxiFocus** - Contains high levels of key carotenoids lutein and zeaxanthin, together with 22 vitamin and minerals identified in a major study as being essential for eye health. Take 4 sprays x 3 times per day for the first three bottles and then reduce to 2 sprays, 3 times per day.

- **Krill Miracle** - Contains Omega 3, 6, and 9 oils that support protection of cell membranes and stabilization of blood sugar levels. Take 1 capsule, 2 times daily.

- **Astaxanthin** -- Powerful biological antioxidant that supports and maintains healthy eyes. Take 2 capsules, 2 times a day.

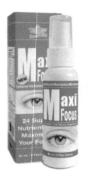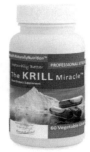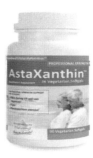

# 2. Supplement Missing Nutrients

- **MaxiFocus** - Contains high levels of key carotenoids lutein and zeaxanthin, together with 22 vitamin and minerals identified in a major study as being essential for eye health. Take 4 sprays x 3 times per day for the first three bottles and then reduce to 2 sprays, 3 times per day.

- **Krill Miracle** - Contains Omega 3, 6, and 9 oils that support protection of cell membranes and stabilization of blood sugar levels. Take 1 capsule, 2 times daily.

- **Astaxanthin** -- Powerful biological antioxidant that supports and maintains healthy eyes. Take 2 capsules, 2 times a day.

- **Active Life** - Delivers a full spectrum of liquid, highly-absorbable multivitamins and minerals. Take 15ml x 2 times daily.

- **Taurine Spray** - Reduces oxidative damage to the eyes and delivers nutrients to the retinal cells, along with assisting in the clean-up of removal products. Take 5 sprays under the tongue daily.

- **Camu Camu** - Provides powerful support to increase energy and maintain the protein collagen of tissues, helping them to heal. Take 1 capsule x 2 times a day.

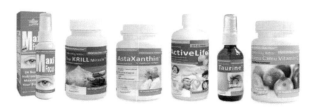

Please note that recommended products and prices may vary and be subject to change, depending on stock level and manufacturer availability.

# 3. Boost the Immune System

- **MaxiFocus** - Contains high levels of key carotenoids lutein and zeaxanthin, together with 22 vitamin and minerals identified in a major study as being essential for eye health. Take 4 sprays x 3 times per day for the first three bottles and then reduce to 2 sprays, 3 times per day.

- **Krill Miracle** - Contains Omega 3, 6, and 9 oils that support protection of cell membranes and stabilization of blood sugar levels. Take 1 capsule, 2 times daily.

- **Astaxanthin** -- Powerful biological antioxidant that supports and maintains healthy eyes. Take 2 capsules, 2 times a day.

- **Active Life** - Delivers a full spectrum of liquid, highly-absorbable multivitamins and minerals. Take 15ml x 2 times daily.

- **Taurine Spray** - Reduces oxidative damage to the eyes and delivers nutrients to the retinal cells, along with assisting in the clean-up of removal products. Take 5 sprays under the tongue daily.

- **Camu Camu** - Provides powerful support to increase energy and maintain the protein collagen of tissues, helping them to heal. Take 1 capsule x 2 times a day.

- **Serranol** - Contains Serrapeptase, Curcuminx4000, Ecklonia Cava, and Vitamin D3 to support eye health by providing better eye circulation, as Serrapeptase can clear inflammation. Curcumin contains anti-inflammatory herbs that stimulate glutathione to protect the cells and the tissue from inflammation, while modulating the immune system. Take 2 x 3 times a day before eating, with water. Reduce to 1 x 3 after 1-2 months.

- **Alpha Lipoic Acid R** - Supports eye health and repairs oxidative damage, regenerating other antioxidants. Take 1 capsule, twice a day.

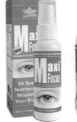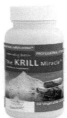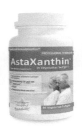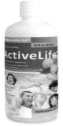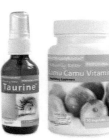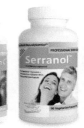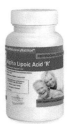

# Optional - But Highly Recommended for At Least 1 to 2 Months

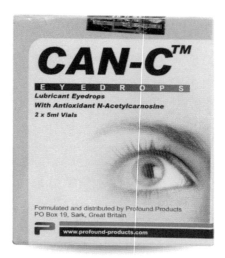

- **CAN-C** - Prevents and reverses cataract development. Take 1-2 drops in each eye, 1-4 times a day.

# 4. Drink More Water.

Drink at least 6-8 glasses of RO filtered or distilled water each day; add a generous pinch of baking soda (sodium bicarbonate) to each glass.

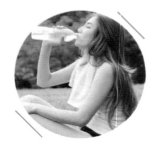

# 5. Cut Out Unnatural, High-Sugar Foods

As the foundation of eye health, cut out starchy carbohydrates altogether, i.e. pastries, cookies, breads, breakfast cereals, pasta, and potatoes, as well as processed foods and milk products.

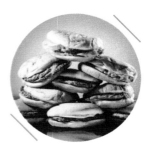

Note: Don't eat turnips, parsnips, and rice, except for small portions of wild rice, brown rice, and sweet potatoes/yams.

# 6. Eat Really Healthy Foods.

## Make sure to eat some of these foods every two hours for the first few months of recovery:

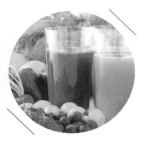

Eat 9-14 servings of fresh or frozen vegetables each day: Try them in soups, steamed, stir-fried, juiced, etc. Eat 50 percent raw, juiced vegetables (preferably organic) and use the pulp to make soup. Blended veggies promote easier digestion.

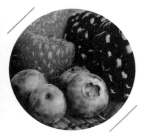

Eat 5 servings of dark-skinned fruits (like cherries, red grapes, blueberries, etc.) that are rich in antioxidants each day.

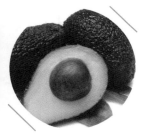

Remember that avocados are a number one superfood with almost a complete spectrum of nutrients. If they are readily available in your area, try to eat at least two a day to promote health recovery. Avocados support heart disease, diabetes, cancer, and eye disease rehabilitation.

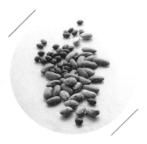

Eat 5 servings of nuts, beans, and seeds (soaked, mashed nuts and seeds).

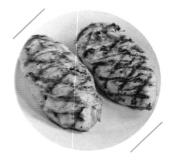

Eat pasture-fed chicken and other meats, only a few servings per week. Grass-fed meat is recommended above corn or grain-fed meat sources.

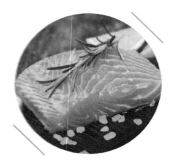

Eat a minimum of 3-4 servings of oily fish each week, if you eat fish. Choose a variety of healthy fish like mackerel, sardines, salmon, etc. Canned fish is a nutritious option, although wild-caught fish is recommended.

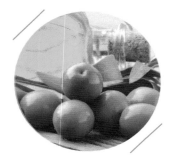

Add healthy oils to your favorite foods, like krill, omega 3, hemp, coconut, and olive oils. Pair with healthy carbohydrate alternatives, like amaranth, quinoa, buckwheat, and chia and millet seeds. You can also try couscous, if you aren't allergic to gluten protein (celiac disease).

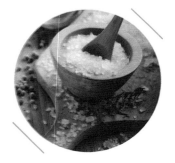

Add 3-5 teaspoons of sea or rock salt, depending on the heat and your body mass, to water or food each day. Remember that sea or rock salt does not contain the important mineral iodine, **so include Nascent Iodine in your rehabilitation plan.**

# Recommended Vegetables

Note: Vegetables may not be available in all countries.

- Artichoke
- Asian Vegetable Sprouts (Wheat, Barley, Alfalfa, etc.)
- Asparagus
- Avocado
- Beetroot
- Broad Beans
- Broccoli
- Brussel Sprouts
- Cabbage (Various Types)
- Capsicum
- Carrots
- Cauliflower
- Celeriac
- Choko
- Cucumber
- Dandelion Leaves
- Dried Peas
- Eggplant (Aubergine)
- Fennel
- Garden Peas
- Garlic
- Kale
- Kohlrabi
- Kumara
- Lettuce (Kos and Various Types)
- Mangetout Peas
- Mushrooms
- Okra
- Onions (Red and White)
- Petit Pois Peas
- Radishes
- Runner Beans
- Seaweed - All Types (Kelp, Wakame, Noni, etc.)
- Silver Beet
- Spinach
- Squash
- Sugar Snap Peas
- Zucchini (Courgettes)

# Recommended Fruits

Note: Fruits may not be available in all countries.

- Apple
- Apricot
- Avocado
- Bilberries
- Blackberries
- Blackcurrants
- Blueberries
- Cherimoya
- Cherries
- Damsons
- Dates
- Durian
- Figs
- Gooseberries
- Grapefruit
- Grapes
- Kiwi Fruit
- Limes
- Lychees
- Mango
- Nectarine
- Orange
- Pear
- Pineapple
- Plum/Prune (Dried Plum)
- Pomegranate
- Rambutan
- Raspberries
- Salal berry
- Satsuma
- Strawberries
- Tangerine
- Western Raspberry (Blackcap)

# The Garden of Eden Pyramid

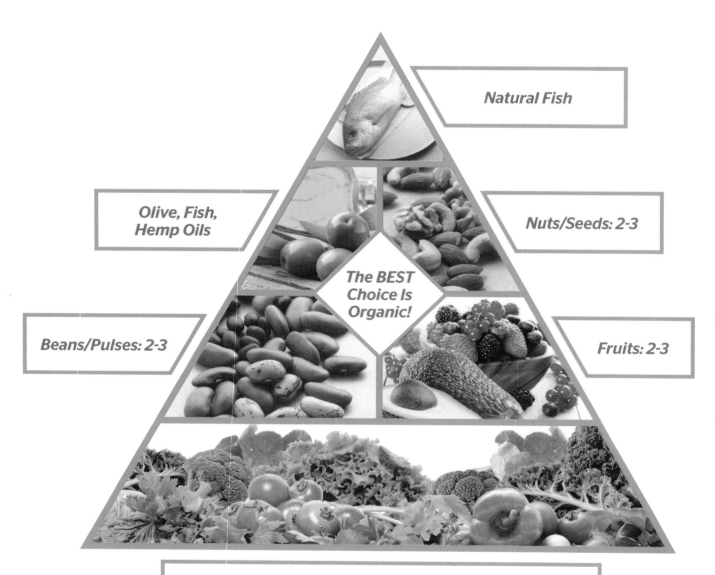

Natural Fish

Olive, Fish, Hemp Oils

Nuts/Seeds: 2-3

The BEST Choice Is Organic!

Beans/Pulses: 2-3

Fruits: 2-3

Vegetables (excluding root): 8-12 servings a day
1/2 raw veggies: Salads, etc.

# 7. Stay Active Daily.

Contrary to the opinion of fitness fanatics, there are two simple ways to get your body working better and stronger. And no, they do not include swimming and cycling, although you can add these later if you want to.

*One of the two simple ways to exercise is to build up to walking 3-5 miles per day, in a fast, purposely strong way with as long a stride as you can. Keep your hands moving from chest level to belt level as you move with each stride.*

*Use weights or wrist weights as you improve.*

*If this is difficult for you at the start, and your lungs are weak, then lie down to exercise to make it easier.*

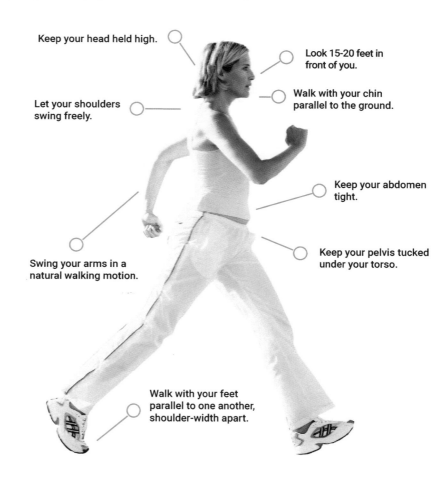

Keep your head held high.

Look 15-20 feet in front of you.

Walk with your chin parallel to the ground.

Let your shoulders swing freely.

Keep your abdomen tight.

Keep your pelvis tucked under your torso.

Swing your arms in a natural walking motion.

Walk with your feet parallel to one another, shoulder-width apart.

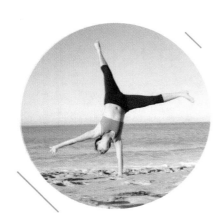

Lie down in a comfortable place. On your bed (if it's firm enough) when you first wake up is a great time and place for this. Bring a knee up to your chest as high as you can get it and then alternate with the other knee. Do as many of these as you can while keeping count. Do this every day and set yourself targets to increase the speed and the number as the weeks go by. You should be doing enough to make your lungs and heart beat faster. At the same time, as you improve your count on your back you need to start walking and build this up.

The second great exercise for strengthening your lungs is to build up slowly where you can exercise at maximum rate for 2 minutes, 6 times per day. It does not matter what exercise you do, e.g. skipping, star jumps, running on the spot; just about anything works, as long as your heart and lungs are working at maximum capacity. By working at maximum rate, your muscles connected with your heart and lungs will get stronger, and health will balance perfectly.

# Physical activity is vital to your rehabilitation plan.

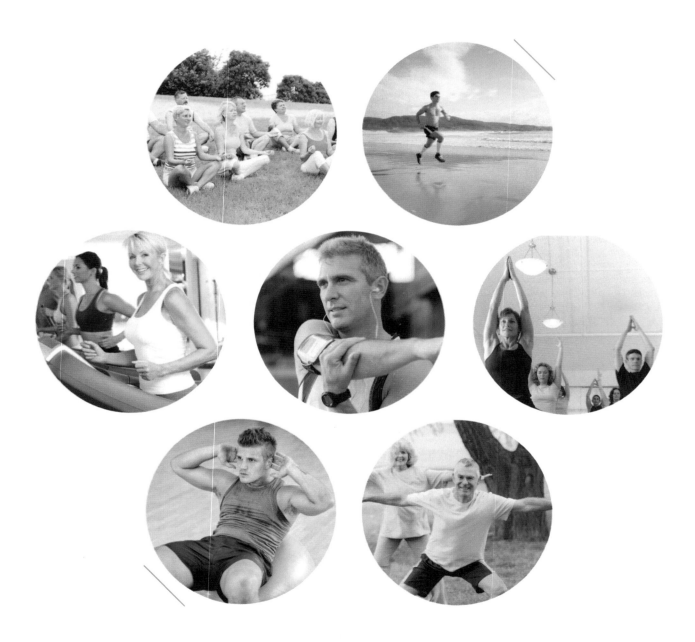

# 8. Learn Proper Breathing

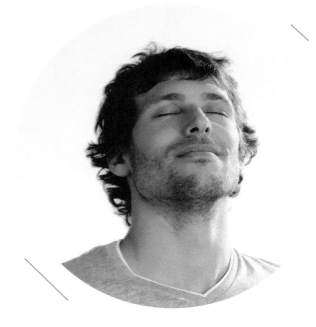 *Breathing properly is critical since oxygen is the foundation of overall health.*

## There are two types of breathing:

1. **Anxious Breathing:** In the chest.
2. **Relaxed Breathing:** In the diaphragm or stomach area.

The first type of breathing in the chest is related to a stress response and includes hormones like cortisol. This stressful breathing should only be temporary since it is related to a fight-or-flight response that causes hormones to release to relax breathing. If stressful breathing grows chronic, the body will retain carbon dioxide and cortisol to affect healthy functioning systems. Stress breathing will also cause the immune system to weaken, leaving it susceptible to infection and disease.

Make it your number one goal to retrain your body to breathe in a relaxed, healthy manner. This will clear out carbon dioxide and cortisol. When carbon dioxide builds up in your bloodstream, it will destroy a substance called hemoglobin that the blood uses to transport oxygen throughout the body. This is why it's especially important to focus on relaxed breathing that comes from the diaphragm.

## How to Breathe Correctly

The easiest way to relearn correct breathing is to lie flat on your back on the floor, on a mat or blanket, or on a firm bed. Place a small weighted object on your belly button, like a heavy book. Take a deep breath in through your nose so that the book rises as your stomach, or diaphragm, fills with air. Hold this deep breath for a count of 4 and then release through your nose so that your stomach deflates. Use this process to release any tension as you exhale and repeat. In the exercise, your chest should not move to indicate relaxed, stress-free breathing.

Practice this low-stress breathing exercise again and again as you lie down. Once you have mastered the rhythm of the calming breath, you can start to try the exercise while standing. Initially, you may feel dizzy as you intake more and more fresh oxygen, but it's still important to practice the exercise whenever you can.

# 9. Stimulate Acupressure Points

Another component in your rehabilitation plan is to stimulate acupressure points that connect to your eye health recovery system. There are a number of points that can be massaged gently with a finger to mimic actual acupuncture. Please read more about this on **page 44.**

# 10. Get More Sun Exposure

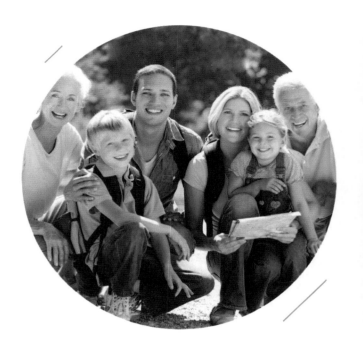

An essential vitamin to support your overall health is vitamin D3. You can find a large dose of vitamin D3 in the recommended supplement on **page 43,** but it's still critical to get some natural vitamin D from sun exposure.

The sun is the source of life. Unfortunately, myths have been circulated in the health community that the sun is an enemy that we must stay away from at all costs. Even worse, many health professionals recommend slathering your body in toxic chemicals every time you go out in the sun. Of course, I'm not recommending lying in the sun for six hours at once on the first hot day of the year. It's essential to build up the skin's tolerance to sun exposure over several weeks for natural protection. By the time that hot summer days come around, you will be able to tolerate a greater amount of natural sun exposure.

---

## Recommendations for sun exposure:

- Expose as much skin as you can to the sun each day, such as on your morning walk.

- Build up your sun exposure gradually from spring to summer seasons.

- Try to stay out of the sun in mid-day without a cover-up; a cover-up is preferred to sunscreen.

- If you do use sunscreen or sun cream, purchase organic products instead of chemical-based, name-brand creams.

- It's important to remember that the sun is your friend, and sunshine can be enjoyed in moderation!

## More About Clearing Inflammation and Promoting Healing

# MaxiFocus

**MaxiFocus** contains high levels of key carotenoids lutein and zeaxanthin, together with 22 vitamins and minerals identified in a major study as being essential for eye health. Presently, we are witnessing a breakthrough in helping to prevent vision loss. MaxiFocus is the *only* sublingual formula delivering this complete spectrum of eye nutrients. These nutrients absorb at least 900 percent better than their tablet equivalent and, in most cases, will be in the eye within **two minutes.**

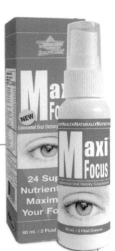

**Ingredients:**

- Vitamin A (as retinyl palmitate) - 5000 IU
- Vitamin D (as colecalciferol) - 400 IU
- Vitamin E (as tocopheryl acetate) - 30 IU
- Thiamin (as thiamin HCL) - 1.5 mg
- Riboflavin (Vitamin B2) - 1.7 mg
- Niacin (as niacinamide) - 5.0 mg
- Vitamin B6 (as pyridoxine HCL) - 2.0 mg
- Folic Acid - 200 mcg
- Vitamin B12 (as methylcobalamin) - 6 mcg
- Biotin - 150 mcg
- Pantothenic acid (as calcium pantothenate) - 10 mg
- Iodine (as potassium iodide) - 152mcg
- Magnesium (as magnesium citrate) - 3.0 mg
- Zinc (as zinc citrate) - 5.0 mg
- Selenium (as sodium selenite) - 55 mcg
- Copper (as copper aspartate) - 0.45 mg
- Chromium (as chromium niacinate) - 30 mcg
- Phosphatidylserine Extract - 20 mg
- Trimethylglycine - 20 mg
- Lutein Extract - 10.0 mg
- L-Taurine - 5.0 mg
- Bilberry Extract - 5.0 mg
- Optisharp® (Zeaxanthin extract) - 2.5 mg
- Ginkgo Biloba Extract - 1.0 mg

**Dosage:**
Take 4 sprays x 3 times per day for the first three bottles and then reduce to 2 sprays, 3 times per day.

# The Krill Miracle

**The Krill Miracle** contains Omega 3, 6, and 9 oils that support protection of cell membranes and stabilization of blood sugar levels.

Krill are tiny shrimp-like crustaceans found in the Southern Oceans. The Southern Oceans are the only oceans in the world that remain unpolluted by the heavy toxic metals that are now found in many fish oils. Krill are a super-rich source of Omega 3, 6, and 9, and their antioxidant levels are 300 times greater than Vitamins A and E and 48 times greater than Omega 3 found in standard fish oils. (Please note: People with seafood allergies should notify their physician prior to taking a krill or fish dietary supplement.)

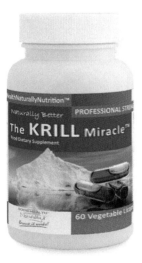

**Ingredients:**

- Superba™ Krill Oil – 1000mg
- Phospholipids – 450mg
- Total Omega 3 – 250mg
- EPA – 120mg
- DHA – 70mg
- Omega 6 – 15mg
- Omega 9 – 80mg
- Astaxanthin - 110µg

**Dosage:**
Take 1 capsule, 2 times daily.

# AstaXanthin with DHA

Strong sunlight, toxins, starchy carbohydrates, lack of fruit and vegetables, and modern living are creating huge amounts of free radical oxidation in our bodies. Only eating 12-14 portions of fruits and vegetables can provide enough antioxidants to clear these free radicals.

**AstaXanthin with DHA** is a naturally occurring carotenoid pigment which is a powerful biological antioxidant. Our product is made using AstaReal Astaxanthin, the most studied astaxanthin in the world with over 50 published studies. It was the first source of astaxanthin for human nutrition reviewed by the U.S. Food and Drug Administration (FDA).

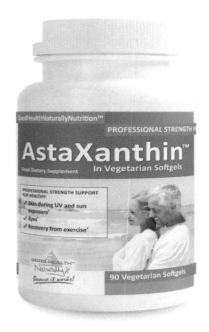

**Ingredients:**

- DHA oil – 180mg
- AstaReal® Astaxanthin 10% - 12mg

**Dosage:**
Take 2 capsules, 2 times a day.

## More About Missing Nutrients

# Active Life

**Active Life - A Daily Dose Of Liquid Vitamins And Minerals** is a liquid formula to ensure you get all the essential vitamins and minerals needed by your body. This single liquid supplement allows for maximum absorption and utilization of the body—300 percent more absorbent than tablets!

| Ingredients: | Amount per Serving: |
|---|---|
| • Calories | 39 |
| • Calcium  (Tricalcium Phosphate, Citrate) | 600mg |
| • Choline Bitartrate | 25mg |
| • Chromium (Chromium Polynicotinate) | 200mcg |
| • Copper (Copper Gluconate) | 2mg |
| • Folic Acid (Vitamin B Conjugate) | 500mcg |
| • Inositol | 50mg |
| • Magnesium (Citrate Gluconate Concentrate) | 300mg |
| • Manganese (Manganese Gluconate) | 10mg |
| • Organic Seleniumethionine | 200mcg |
| • Potassium (Potassium Gluconate) | 250mg |
| • Vitamin A (Palmitate) | 5000IU |
| • Vitamin A (Beta Carotene) | 5000IU |
| • Vitamin B1 (Thiamine Mononitrate) | 3mg |
| • Vitamin B12 (Methylcobalamin) | 6mcg |
| • Vitamin B2 (Riboflavin) | 3.4mg |
| • Vitamin B3 (Niacinamide) | 40mg |
| • Vitamin B5 (Calcium Pantothenate) | 20mg |
| • Vitamin B6 (Pyridoxine Hydrochloride) | 4mg |
| • Vitamin C (Ascorbic Acid) | 300mg |
| • Vitamin D (Cholecalciferol) | 400IU |
| • Vitamin E (Alpha Tocopheryl Acetate) | 60IU |
| • Vitamin K (Phytonadione) | 80mcg |
| • Zinc (Oxide) | 15mg |
| • Ionic Trace Minerals | 600mg |
| • Phosphorus (Amino Acid Chelate) | 190mg |
| • Biotin | 300mcg |
| • Iodine (Potassium Iodine) | 150mcg |
| • Boron (Sodium Borate) | 2mg |
| • Molybdenum | 75mcg |
| • Chloride Concentrate | 102mg |
| • Amino Acid Complex | 10mg |
| • Aloe Vera Extract (200:1) | 2 mg |

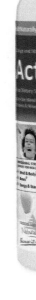

**Dosage:**
Take 15ml x 2 times daily.

**Allergen Info:** Contains Corn. GLUTEN FREE.

# Taurine Spray

**Taurine** is an amino acid from protein, found in high levels in the retina, and is thought to protect against both ultraviolet light and toxic substances. Taurine Spray contains the same natural ingredient and is therefore thought to nourish and defend against damage from UV light (thereby protecting against macular degeneration).

Taurine is depleted in diabetics, which raises the question of whether its deficiency contributes to the development of diabetic retinopathy as well as to other complications of diabetes. It is suspected, but not proved, that taurine deficiency may contribute to the development of age-related macular degeneration, and hence, logical supplementation with taurine may help to protect against it.

# Camu Camu

**Camu Camu** provides powerful support to increase energy and maintain the protein collagen of tissues, helping them to heal. Camu Camu fruit has one of the highest recorded amounts of natural vitamin C, providing over 2,700 mg of vitamin C per 100 grams of fruit. It is rich in vitamins, minerals, and complex amino acids that aid in the absorption of vitamin C; it is an excellent source of potassium, providing more than 700 mg per kg of fruit!

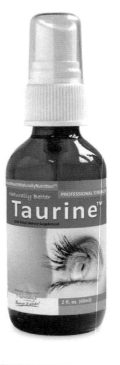

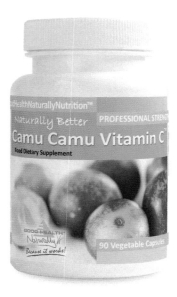

**Ingredients:**
- L-Taurine – 50mg

**Dosage:**
Take 5 sprays under the tongue daily.

**Ingredients:**
- Natural Vitamin C (from Camu Camu Powder) – 105mg
- Camu Camu Extract 15% - 700mg

**Dosage:**
Take 1 capsule, 2 times a day.

## More About Immune Strengthening Formulations

# Super Nutrient Serranol™

Super Nutrient Serranol™ offers professional strength support for healthy joints, cells, heart, blood flow, circulation, and cholesterol with ingredients like:

- **Serrapeptidase** (technically Serriatia Peptidase) is a multi-functional proteolytic enzyme that dissolves non-living tissues, such as scarring, fibrin, plaque, blood clots, cysts, and inflammation in all forms—without harming living tissue. Serrapeptidase helps promote better wellbeing for your inflammatory system and supports your whole body, not only the lungs but also arteries, digestive tract, colon, joints, and anywhere blockages/ inflammation needs resolving.

- **Curcumin (CurcuminX4000)** is one of the best natural anti-inflammatory herbs to stimulate glutathione to protect cells and tissue from inflammation and help modulate the immune system. Curcumin has also been studied for its anti-bacterial, anti-viral, and anti-fungal properties.

- **Ecklonia Cava (Seanol®)** - For centuries, people throughout Asia have consumed Ecklonia Cava Extract, a species of edible brown algae. Harvested from the coastal waters off Japan, Korea, and China, all studies indicate ECE offers outstanding health benefits.

- **Vitamin D3** is critical to keep your immune system strong. The cells that make up the immune system contain vitamin D3 receptors. If there is an insufficient amount of vitamin D3 present to bind receptors, immune cells become weak and cannot protect the body from infections. Vitamin D3 deficiency is increasingly common in people of all ages because we spend less time outdoors in the sun, but this vital vitamin cannot be stored in the body. So replenishment through daily supplementation is vital to immune health.

# Alpha Lipoic Acid R

Alpha Lipoic Acid R supports eye health and repairs oxidative damage, regenerating other antioxidants. Alpha Lipoic Acid is a 'network' antioxidant that provides support for healthy blood sugar levels, peripheral nerves, digestion, glandular activity, and the liver. In addition to neutralizing free radicals, ALA has been studied for its potential abilities in the repair of oxidative damage, regeneration of other antioxidants, anti-inflammatory properties, and chelation of excess metals.

Alpha Lipoic Acid R is significantly more bio-available than the 'free acid' form of R-Lipoic Acid (RLA). In a preliminary trial, the maximum plasma concentration was 40 times higher than that of unstabilized RLA.

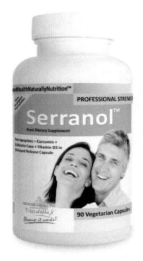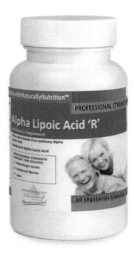

---

**Ingredients:**

- SerraEnzyme Serrapeptase® - 80,000iu
- Curcumin X4000 - 250mg
- Ecklonia Cava Extract (Seanol®) - 50mg
- Vitamin D3 - 1000iu

**Dosage:**
Take 2 x 3 times a day before eating, with water. Reduce to 1 x 3 after 1-2 months.

---

**Ingredients:**

- Bio-enhanced® Na-RALA – 200mg

**Dosage:**
Take 1 capsule, twice a day.

More About Optional Nutrients

# Can-C

**Can-C** prevents and reverses cataract development. Can-C NAC Eye Drops (previously Re-Vital Eyes NAC Drops) is the original, high purity, tested, and approved brand. If you want assurances about what will work and what will be safe in your eye to use for months at a time, *insist* on Can-C Eyes Eye Drops.

N-Acetyl Carnosine drops can be used for lubrication of the eyes and as part of the control of cataracts.

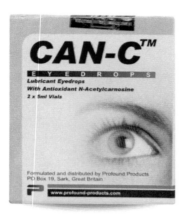

Ingredients:

- N-Acetyl Carnosine (NAC) - 1%
- Glycerin (lubricant) - 1%
- Carboxymethylcellulose sodium (lubricant) - 0.3%

**Dosage:**
Take 1-2 drops in each eye, 1-4 times a day.

# More About Acupressure

Stimulating the Good Health points on pages 11-13 and 8.20-8.21 of the book **Mastering Acupuncture** will help to balance eye health. These points can be effectively and safely stimulated using the **HealthPoint™** electro-acupressure kit. The advantage of the kit is that it gives you the power to precisely locate the acupuncture point, and indeed other points, so you can enjoy the benefits of acupuncture at home and without any needles.

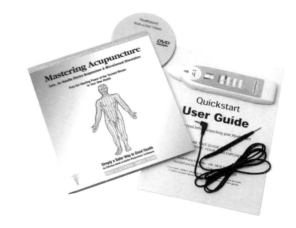

**HealthPoint™** is easy to use, painless, and effective. It includes an instructional DVD and book covering over 150 pain and non-pain conditions that can be helped, such as headaches, back, neck, and joint problems.

The gentle and systematic stimulation of the body's natural healing system can speed recovery in many cases. **HealthPoint™** breakthrough waveform was developed with leading pain control specialist Dr. Julian Kenyon, MD, 21 years ago. Today, it features the latest microchip technology to quickly locate acupuncture points key to specific health conditions, such as the points for eye disease recovery.

# Electro-Acupressure Heals Eye Disease?

## Acupuncture Protocol For Treatment Of Age-Related Macular Degeneration by Dr. Alston C. Lundgren

For those with age-related macular degeneration, electro-acupressure has a special importance. While acupuncture has been used for thousands of years to increase circulation to the eyes and provide relief for strain, fatigue, irritation, and blurred vision, research supports acupuncture to treat ARMD.

In a study conducted on 108 patients, 56 women and 52 men with an age range of 47 to 96 years old, acupuncture treatment was used in a combination of ear acupuncture, periorbital electrical stimulation, and a French Energetic technique. In the study group, all patients had been diagnosed by an ophthalmologist with macular degeneration.

Following the treatment, 69 percent of patients improved in distant vision and 69 percent improved in near vision. Patients with both wet and dry ARMD saw the same improvements. Up to 7 percent of patients saw an improvement in color vision. Researchers noted that, "Visual acuity in [ARMD] may be improved by acupuncture."

In *The Body Electric*, Robert Becker illustrates the importance of microcurrent stimulation acupressure as a means to heal the body. Becker discovered that voltage differences may appear in the body following injury or disease. An injury can create a positive charge in an affected area, thus serving as a bioelectric battery that needs to be "turned on." Research supports microcurrent stimulation to heal the body, with special benefits for eye health.

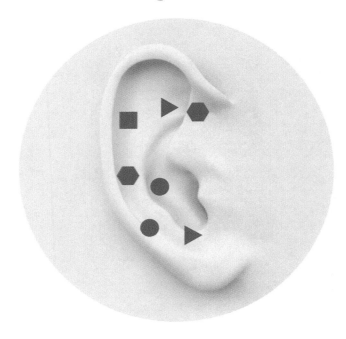

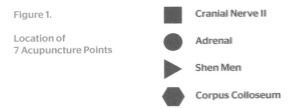

Figure 1.

Location of 7 Acupuncture Points

■ Cranial Nerve II

● Adrenal

▶ Shen Men

⬡ Corpus Colloseum

*Source: The American Academy of Medical Acupuncture [AAMA], Publisher of the journal Medical Acupuncture, Volume 16, Number 3, May 2005.*

## In Conclusion:

The Eye Disease Rehabilitation Program offers a complete plan that is specially designed to comprehensively prevent or manage debilitating eye disease.

Eye disease can better be understood as a lifestyle disease. This means that if you change your lifestyle, there is a greater chance of partial or full recovery. When you implement the changes found in the 10 Step Plan, your body can naturally begin the healing process to recover your vision.

### 👁 *Drugs won't improve your health.*

Drugs aren't effective since they can't make you healthy again. In a best-case scenario, drugs may provide some relief. In a worst-case scenario, they will further damage your health and can even cause untimely death.

Of course, the pharmaceutical industry would love you to continue on your current drug regimen and ineffective rehabilitation plan, relying on toxic medications that inhibit your true path to long-term healing.

### 👁 *Thankfully, you have discovered that there is a better way.*

**The care of your body requires a complete program, one designed to address all aspects of what is needed to regain your eyesight:**

- The Eye Disease Rehabilitation Program is structured for ill patients with chronic problems whose quality of life has decreased, even after receiving medical treatment.

- This program can help you learn how to take a deep breath, relax, and improve your quality of life. The program includes treatment, exercise training, education, and coaching.

- This personalized program incorporates therapy, support, and education to assist you in achieving the best eye health possible, based on your specific condition.

You will find the Eye Disease Rehabilitation Program outlined in this book. When you follow it carefully, you will see some results starting within weeks.

### 👁 *This rehabilitation plan will always offer health improvements.*

The worst outcome when using this plan will be that your health improves, but you still need to take some drugs if your eye health has been damaged irreparably by medication or disease.

### 👁 *Start slowly and begin rehabilitation step-by-step.*

If you're not used to making major changes in your life, it may be difficult to adopt new healthy habits at first. But stick with it because...

### 👁 *Your health is invaluable...*

Robert Redfern, Your Health Coach

Email: robert@goodhealth.nu
www.MyGoodHealthClub.com
for step-by-step coaching and support.

# Daily Healthy Vision Rehabilitation Plan

| TIME | ACTION | AMOUNT |
| --- | --- | --- |
| **OPTIONAL ITEMS** | | |
| Various times throughout the day | Can-C | Take 1-2 drops in each eye, 1-4 times a day |
| **BREAKFAST** | | |
| 30 minutes before breakfast | Serranol | Take 2 capsules, with water |
| With breakfast | MaxiFocus | Take 4 sprays |
| With breakfast | Active Life | Take 15ml with water |
| With breakfast | Krill Miracle | Take 1 capsule |
| With breakfast | Taurine Spray | Take 5 sprays under the tongue |
| With breakfast | Alpha Lipoic Acid R | Take 1 capsule |
| With breakfast | Camu Camu | Take 1 capsule |
| **LUNCH** | | |
| 30 minutes before lunch | Serranol | Take 2 capsules, with water |
| With lunch | MaxiFocus | Take 4 sprays |
| With lunch | AstaXanthin with DHA | Take 2 capsules |
| With lunch | Active Life | Take 15ml with water |
| With lunch | Alpha Lipoic Acid R | Take 1 capsule |
| **EVENING MEAL** | | |
| 30 minutes before evening meal | Serranol | Take 2 capsules, with water |
| With your evening meal | MaxiFocus | Take 4 sprays |
| With your evening meal | Krill Miracle | Take 1 capsule |
| With your evening meal | AstaXanthin with DHA | Take 2 capsules |
| With your evening meal | Camu Camu | Take 1 capsule |

## References

1. 1 Bausch + Lomb Global Barometer of Eye Health, 2012.

2. Barnard, Neal D. *Nutrition Guide for Clinicians*. Washington, DC: PCRM/Physicians Committee for Responsible Medicine, 2009. Print.

3. "Retina." *Wikipedia*. Wikimedia Foundation.

4. "Central Vision Definition - Medical Dictionary Definitions of Popular Medical Terms Easily Defined on MedTerms." *Medterms*.

5. Ganea E, Harding JJ. "Result Filters." *National Center for Biotechnology Information*. U.S. National Library of Medicine.

6. A.D.A.M. Medical Encyclopedia.

7. Vasireddy et al. "Rescue of Photoreceptor Degeneration by Curcumin in Transgenic Rats with P23H Rhodopsin Mutation." *PLoS ONE, June 2011, vol. 6(6), pp. e21193.*

8. Petri D, Lundebye AK. *Comp Biochem Physiol C Toxicol Pharmacol. 2007 Mar; 145(2):202-9.*

9. "Cytotoxic effects of curcumin in human retinal pigment epithelial cells." *PLoS One. 2013; 8(3): e59603.*

10. Dagnelie G., et al *Optometry 2000 Mar;71(3):147-64.*

11. JM Seddon et al. *1994 Journal of the American Medical Association 272:1420.*

12. Age-Related Eye Disease Study Research Group, The Relationship of Dietary Arytenoids and Vitamin A, E and C.

13. Head KA, *Altern Med Rev 1999 Oct;4(5):342-59.*

14. KJ Yeum et al. *1995 Investigative Ophthalmology & Visual Science 36:2756-61.*

15. Landrum, et al. *Exp Eye Res 1997 Jul;65(1):57-62*

16. "Glutathione: The Eye Healer Within." *Glutathione: The Eye Healer Within.*

17. Lundgren, AC. *An acupuncture protocol for treatment of age-related macular degeneration: A second report.*

## Recommended Books:

- **Cancer Cell Rehabilitation in 30 Days**

- **Solving Diabetes Type 2 in 27 Days**

- **Improving Arthritis in 30 Days**

- **Improving Multiple Sclerosis in 30 Days**

- **Improving Candida in 30 Days**

- **Improving Heart Disease in 30 Days**

- **Improving Lung Health in 30 Days**

- **Improving Kidney Health in 30 Days**

## Other Books by Robert Redfern:

- *The 'Miracle Enzyme' Is Serrapeptase*

- *Turning a Blind Eye*

- *Mastering Acupuncture*

- *EquiHealth Equine Acupressure*

_____

_____

_____

_____

_____

_____

_____

_____

_____

_____

_____

_____

_____

_____

_____

_____

_____

_____

_____

_____

_____

Made in the USA
Lexington, KY
14 February 2017